THE WEIGHT -LOSS CURE

How to Fight Cravings, Attain Energy, and Slim Down

By

Kenneth. N. Ashford

Table of Content:

Chapter 5: **Obesity Solution Meal: How to Fight Sugar Cravings and Choose the Right Macronutrients**
- Macronutrients and Weight: Do Carbs, Protein, or Fat Matter?
- Beyond Willpower: Diet Quality and Quantity Matter

Chapter six: **Healthy Nutritional Supplements**

Introduction

Many factors influence body weight genes, though the effect is small, and heredity is not destiny; prenatal and early life influences; poor diets; too much television watching; too little physical activity and sleep; and our food and physical activity environment.

The causes of obesity are as varied as the people it affects. These results when someone regularly takes in more calories than needed. The body stores these excess calories as fat, and over-time pounds add up. Eat fewer calories than the body burns whiles fat goes down.

This equation can be deceptively simple, though, because it doesn't account for the number of factors that affect what we eat, how much we exercise, and how our bodies process all this energy. A complex web surrounds a simple problem. The Obesity Solution shows you how to become the master of your body and lose fat rather than recommending a specific diet or restricting others.

CHAPTER 1

What Results in the Scales of Excess Fatness?

The causes of obesity are as varied as the people it affects. Obesity results when someone regularly takes in more calories than needed. The body stores these excess calories as body fat, and over time the extra pounds add up. Eat fewer calories than the body burns, weight goes down. This equation can be deceptively simple, though, because it doesn't account for the multitude of factors that affect what we eat, how much we exercise, and how our bodies process all this energy. A complex web surrounds a basic problem.

What are some of the factors that increase the risk of obesity?

Genes Are Not Destiny

Heredity plays a role in obesity but generally to a much lesser degree than many people might believe.

Rather than being obesity's sole cause, genes seem to increase the risk of weight gain and interact with other risk factors in the environment, such as unhealthy diets and inactive lifestyles.

And healthy lifestyles can counteract these genetic effects. Genes influence every aspect of human physiology, development, and adaptation. Obesity is no exception. Yet relatively little is known regarding the specific genes that contribute to obesity the scale of so-called "genetic environment interactions" and the complex interplay between our genetic makeup and our life experiences.

Prenatal and Postnatal Influences

The Weight-Loss Cure

Early life is important, too. Pregnant mothers who smoke or who are overweight may have children who are more likely to grow up to be obese adults. Excessive weight gain during infancy also raises the risk of adult obesity, while being breastfed may lower the risk.

Obesity, once thought to be little more than an unfortunate failure of will and self-restraint, has much deeper and more complex roots. Genes play a role in driving an individual's propensity to gain excess weight, as do the environment and gene-environment interactions. Early-life influences, beginning with the intrauterine environment and continuing through the first few years of life, also shape the trajectory of weight gain and body fatness throughout the life course.

Later data showing that higher birth weight is also associated with obesity, diabetes, and other adult diseases has helped extend this concept into the "developmental origins hypothesis," which encompasses the preconception period as well as many critical periods of fetal and infant development. During each of these periods, several factors appear to have a substantial impact on obesity in childhood and adulthood. This article briefly outlines some of the key prenatal and early life influences on the development of adult weight and obesity. In the 1980s, intriguing research from British epidemiologist David Barker and colleagues sparked a flutter of research into what was then called the "fatal origins hypothesis" of chronic disease. They proposed that coronary heart disease, type 2 diabetes, stroke, hypertension, and other chronic diseases develop in part due to undernutrition during fetal life and infancy.

The warm, nutrient- and hormone-rich environment of the uterus has a profound effect on fetal development. Brief or fluctuating changes in the intrauterine environment at critical or sensitive periods of the developmental process, as well as longer-term alterations, could have irreversible, lifelong consequences. Three modifiable prenatal factors that appear to shape fatal nutrition and health in later life are

the mother's smoking habits during pregnancy; Although smoking during pregnancy tends to slow the rate of fatal growth, children of women who smoke during pregnancy are more likely to be obese than the children of women who don't. In a meta-analysis of 14 studies, maternal smoking during pregnancy was associated with a 50 percent higher risk of childhood obesity. Most of the studies looked at children's obesity status at ages 3 to 7; one study assessed obesity at age 14, and another tracked the children to young adulthood.

· the mother's weight gain during pregnancy; and Excessive weight gain during pregnancy is more common now than it was in 1990 when the Institute of Medicine (IOM) first offered recommendations for pregnancy-related weight gain. In addition, more women are beginning pregnancy overweight or obese. These worrisome changes prompted the IOM to re-evaluate what constitutes healthy weight gain during pregnancy, with new evidence suggesting that weight gain once considered normal by the IOM increases the risk of childhood obesity.

Project Viva, for example, is a Boston-area study that began following more than 2,000 pregnant women and their offspring soon after the women discovered they were pregnant, and it will continue following the women and children at least through early adolescence. Using data from this cohort, investigators looked at the relationship between a mother's weight gain during pregnancy, defined by the 1990 IOM guidelines, and her child's risk of obesity at age 3.

Children of women who gained an "excessive" amount of weight had more than four times the risk of being overweight at age 3, compared with children of women who gained an "inadequate" amount of weight. Even women who gained what was considered at the time to be an "adequate" amount of weight bore children who were nearly four times more likely to be overweight at age 3 than children of women who gained an "inadequate" amount of weight.

· **the mother's blood sugar level during pregnancy, specifically, whether she develops pregnancy-related (gestational) diabetes.**

It makes intuitive sense that the mother's diet during pregnancy should also affect fetal development and birth weight, but evidence for this is inconsistent.

Weight gain during pregnancy is primarily adipose (fat) tissue. The proliferation of adipose tissue is often accompanied by a state of relative insulin resistance starting in mid-pregnancy. This adaptive response allows for more efficient transfer of glucose and other fuels across the placenta, so the foetus can grow. However, it may also subject the fetus to periods of high blood glucose and elevated insulin. These can lead to increased body fat, which generally manifests as larger size at birth. Many studies show that birth weight is directly associated with later BMI, so it makes sense that gestational diabetes in a mother may contribute to obesity in her child.

Indeed, among 5- to 7-year-old children in two American health plans, the risk of having a high weight for their age was increased among those whose mothers had untreated gestational diabetes, compared with children whose mothers did not have diabetes. Among children whose mothers received treatment for gestational diabetes, the risk was lower, about equal to that of children whose mothers had less severe glucose intolerance.

Although these data suggest that treatment of gestational diabetes could lower the risk of childhood obesity, a more recent study of 4- to 5-year-old children whose mothers participated in a gestational diabetes treatment trial found no difference in obesity rates between children of women who received treatment for mild gestational diabetes and children of women who did not. The jury is still out on the extent to which gestational diabetes causes childhood obesity, but preventing and treating gestational diabetes benefits the baby in other ways.

Unhealthy Diets

What's become the typical Western diet-frequent, large meals high in refined grains, red meat, unhealthy fats, and sugary drinks play one of the largest roles in obesity. Foods that are lacking in the Western whole grains, vegetables, fruits, and nuts seem to help with weight control and also help prevent chronic disease.

An unhealthy diet refers to a pattern of eating that includes excessive consumption of processed foods, high levels of added sugars, unhealthy fats, and insufficient intake of essential nutrients. It often involves the overconsumption of calorie-dense but nutrient-poor foods such as fast food, sugary beverages, and snacks.

Impact of an Unhealthy Diet

- **Obesity and Weight Gain:** One of the most noticeable impacts of an unhealthy diet is weight gain and obesity. Consuming excessive calories without adequate nutrient content leads to the accumulation of body fat, resulting in a higher risk of obesity-related health conditions like diabetes, high blood pressure, and certain types of cancer.
- **Nutritional Deficiencies:** Unhealthy diets often lack the necessary vitamins, minerals, and antioxidants needed for optimal health. This deficiency can lead to weakened immune systems, fatigue, poor concentration, and an increased susceptibility to illnesses.
- **Increased Risk of Chronic Diseases:** A diet high in processed foods, unhealthy fats, and added sugars contributes to an increased risk of chronic diseases such as heart disease,

stroke, and certain types of cancer. These foods are typically low in essential nutrients and contain harmful additives that can harm our cardiovascular system and overall health.

- **Mental Health Issues:** Research suggests a strong connection between unhealthy diets and mental health issues such as depression and anxiety. Nutrient deficiencies and the presence of harmful substances in processed foods can negatively affect brain function and mood regulation.

Why Do People Follow Unhealthy Diets?

Several factors contribute to the prevalence of unhealthy diets among individuals. Here are some common reasons:

- **Convenience:** In our fast-paced world, processed and fast foods offer convenience and time-saving options. However, these foods often lack nutritional value and tend to be high in unhealthy fats, sodium, and sugars.
- **Emotional Eating:** Many individuals turn to food as a coping mechanism for stress, anxiety, or other emotional triggers. Unfortunately, these comfort foods are typically unhealthy and provide temporary relief while harming long-term health.
- **Lack of Nutrition Education:** Limited knowledge about nutrition and healthy eating practices can lead people to make poor dietary choices. Without understanding the importance of balanced meals, they may rely on convenience foods or fad diets.
- **Advertising and Marketing:** Aggressive advertising and marketing campaigns by the food industry often promote unhealthy products, making them appear attractive and appealing to consumers.

Too Much Television, Too Little Activity, and Too Little Sleep

The Weight-Loss Cure

Television watching is a strong obesity risk factor, in part because exposure to food and beverage advertising can influence what people eat. Physical activity can protect against weight gain, but globally, people just aren't doing enough of it. Lack of sleep hallmark of the Western lifestyle also emerging as a risk factor for obesity.

The epidemic nature of obesity in industrialized countries is a serious health and social concern. The number of obese people has significantly increased in the past 20 years. In Poland, excess weight and obesity are a serious epidemiological concern. In terms of the number of overweight people, Poland is a leader in Europe. Therefore, indicating many serious health concerns that are the natural consequences of this phenomenon has become important from the point of view of public health. This work identifies numerous diseases that are a direct consequence of obesity due to bad eating habits and lack of physical exercise among Poles. It discusses the negative effect of television and food commercials contributing to an increase in obesity, not only among adults but also among children. This is an overview forming grounds for further studies into ways of preventing the development of diseases due to obesity, both in Poland and in the world

Toxic Environment-Food and Physical Activity

As key as individual choices are when it comes to health, no one person behaves in a vacuum. The physical and social environment in which people live plays a huge role in the food and activity choices they make. And, unfortunately, in the U.S. and increasingly around the globe, this environment has become toxic to healthy living: The incessant and unavoidable marketing of unhealthy foods and sugary drinks. The lack of safe areas for exercising. The junk food is sold at school, at work, and the corner store. Add it up, and it's tough for individuals to make the healthy choices that are so important to a good quality of life and a healthy weight.

Obesity and its causes have, in many ways, become woven into the fabric of our society. To successfully disentangle them will take a multifaceted approach that not only gives individuals the skills to make healthier choices but also sets in place policies and infrastructure that support those choices.

What we choose to eat plays a large role in determining our risk of gaining too much weight. But our choices are shaped by the complex world in which we live the kinds of food our parents make available at home, by how far we live from the nearest supermarket or fast food restaurant, and even by the ways that governments support farmers. In the U.S. and many parts of the world, the so-called food environment physical and social surroundings that influence what we eat make it far too hard to choose healthy foods, and all too easy to choose unhealthy foods. Some even call this food environment "toxic" because of the way it corrodes healthy lifestyles and promotes obesity.

Food Environment Research by Setting

Families

Families influence children's dietary choices and risk of obesity in several ways, and children develop food preferences at home that can last well into adulthood.

The food that families keep at home and how family members share meals influences what and how much they eat. Not surprisingly, a recent review of published studies found a strong association between the availability of fruits and vegetables at home and whether children, adolescents, and adults eat these foods. Eating meals as a family has also been linked with increased child and adolescent intake of fruit vegetables and other healthy foods. Increased frequency of family meals has been linked with lower BMI in some studies but not in others.

Low-income families face additional barriers to healthy eating that may contribute to the higher rates of obesity seen in lower-income groups. One roadblock is that healthy foods, such as vegetables, fruits, and whole grains, are more expensive than less healthful foods, such as refined grains and sweets, and may be too expensive for low-income families. Another is time: It takes longer to prepare healthful meals than to buy convenience foods or fast food. But people in lower-income households, often single parents working full time and taking care of children, may have less time for meal preparation and other household chores.

Worksites

Employed adults in the U.S. spend about one-quarter of all of their time at work. Worksites often provide easy access to unhealthy foods in vending machines and limited access to healthier options, such as fruits and vegetables. Several studies have shown that making changes to the workplace food environment, such as offering more healthy foods in company cafeterias, results in improved diet quality.

Work environments can also increase the risk of obesity arising from job stress and work-related fatigue, which are linked to poor diets and reduced physical activity. Time at work also plays a role: Shift workers and employees working longer-than-usual hours every week have a higher risk of obesity.

Schools

The Weight-Loss Cure

Just as employed adults spend most of their day at work, children spend much of their day at school. In the U.S., the National School Lunch Program and related federal school meal programs, administered by the U.S. Department of Agriculture, serve more than 30 million children every day, including breakfast, lunch, and after-school snacks. Researchers have found that participating in the School Breakfast Program is associated with lower BMI in children, while participating in the lunch program did not affect obesity. Students participating in the School Breakfast Program were also less likely to skip breakfast, which may reduce the risk of being overweight by spreading food intake more evenly across the day.

Most schools sell food to students outside of the school meal programs. These so-called "competitive foods" are widely available in the cafeteria, vending machines, and school stores. In 2004-2005, 40 percent of all U.S. students ate competitive foods on a given school day, mostly foods high in calories and low in nutritional value, otherwise known as junk food. Eating competitive foods has been linked with poorer quality diets and an increased risk of obesity in several studies.

In addition to unhealthy foods, schools have long provided a ready supply of sugar-sweetened beverages, which are linked to increased risk of obesity and diabetes. Although recent agreements between the Alliance for a Healthier Generation and the American Beverage Association have substantially reduced the supply of sugary beverages, schools continue to offer students unhealthy sugar-sweetened beverages. But policies that curb access to sugary drinks on school property could be a promising strategy for helping children cut back: Boston banned sugary drinks in public schools in 2004, and researchers found that after the policy change took place, city students cut back, overall, on sugary drinks.

Neighborhoods

People will have a hard time eating healthfully if healthy foods just aren't available where they live. Several aspects of the neighborhood food environment have drawn research attention, chief among them, how the presence or lack of nearby supermarkets, convenience stores, and fast-food restaurants relates to obesity risk. Researchers have also looked at whether economic and racial/ethnic disparities in neighborhood food environments may, in part, explain the higher rates of obesity found in individuals who have lower socioeconomic status (lower incomes, education, and job status), and in Blacks and Hispanics in the U.S.

CHAPTER 2

The Energy Unit Problem (Caloric Principles) Does binge eating inevitably result in weight gain?

A calorie is a unit of energy equating to approximately 4.1868 joules of energy and is loosely defined as the amount of heat needed to raise the temperature of a quantity of water by one degree.

All nutritive foods contain calories and our ability to convert that energy into another usable form of energy within the body is the reason (quite simply) that we are alive and the reason our bodies can perform all physical and physiological tasks, including breathing, digesting food, thinking, and moving.

The amount of energy foods provide is normally recorded in thousands of calories (kilocalories or kcal). However, people often use the term "calories" instead, since "kilocalories" is an awkward word to use!

What are the pitfalls of counting calories?

There are many reasons why you may wish to take a long hard look at calorie counting as a strategy for achieving your goals or improving your health circumstances (including HA recovery). I've summarized some of the key considerations below.

Human bodies are not laboratories

The idea that a calorie "*is a calorie, is a calorie*" is so pervasive that we often forget about the sources of these calories, the context in which they are found, and how they are used in the body.

You've probably heard the phrase "All calories are equal". Yet whilst calories may be "equal" outside the body, this is not the case inside the body. The actual energy (or "calorie") content of certain foods may differ from the energy that is theoretically calculated and this is due to key differences in food digestibility and food structure. It follows that when comparing different foods that contain the same number of calories, this does not mean that those foods will affect the body in the same way.

Whilst historically the calorie "system" takes into some consideration the processes involved in the digestion and absorption of calories from different foods and macronutrients, the same cannot be said for the metabolism of those foods. That is, different nutrients contain different biochemical structures that require different biochemical pathways and processes for extracting their energy.

Protein provides a brilliant example of this. Technically, carbohydrates and proteins (gram for gram) share the same caloric "value". Both proteins and carbohydrates contain approximately (note, this value is not definite) 4kcal per gram.

However, the calories in protein are only 70% available for use as energy, once they have been metabolized (the energy "releasing" process that occurs after digestion and absorption). The energy derived from carbohydrates is conversely ~92% available, whilst fats provide ~98% energy (or caloric) availability.

But let's look at another example. Take tree nuts, for example. Nuts are well known for their energy density and high fat content (ranging between 40–75 g per 100 g). However, eating nuts as part of a healthy diet does not affect body weight (and thus energy balance), according to experimental and observational studies.

The reasons for this are proposed to include mechanisms involving appetite control, dietary-induced thermogenesis (how much heat foods release in the process of extracting their energy), and discrepancies in the amount of the "food available energy" to the human body.

So, you see that the composition of one's diet plays a huge role in how accurately and how effectively we can actually "calorie count".

How we prepare and consume food makes a difference

The nuances of food composition and the energy (or caloric) availability of foods are further confounded by how we select, prepare, and consume different foods.

As alluded to above in the case of nuts, the presence of fiber (a group of complex, undigestible carbohydrates found in plants) makes food harder to break down, reducing the accessibility of some of the energy stored in the food. Even natural differences in food state (whether we prefer to eat green or yellow bananas, for example) change the energy availability of the food, to a degree.

Different preparation methods, like cooking, blending, and juicing, also make a difference with industrial processing methods in particular making food more energy "available" to us.

How we "combine" foods also matters. Whether we eat carbohydrates on our own or with proteins, fats, and fiber will affect the glycaemic load (a measurement of how much food will raise a person's blood glucose after eating it). This, in turn, will have an impact on how we use and store that energy.

Counting calories blindly removes the context from which that calorie originated in the food, what effect different foods and their combinations can have on our hormones, and even the brain chemistry that controls hunger and eating behaviors.

Our energy requirements are not uniform or static

As wonderful as it is to feel in control of our health with a daily calorie "quota", generic calorie prescriptions, such as 2000kcal per day for women and 2500kcal per day for men, are based on population averages that may not be relevant or hugely helpful in the context of individual health. We are all quite simply wonderfully (and energetically) unique.

One of the ways this is expressed is in our gut microbiota (the microbial populations that live within our guts). In recent years emerging evidence has shown us that these microbial species have a marked impact on our ability to harvest energy from digested food. Whilst the extent to which we can (and should) influence this internal ecosystem to promote health is not yet fully known, the impact of the microbiota on the calorie "currency" of food will differ from person to person.

Another important consideration is that a daily calorie prescription will not take into account the daily changes in energy requirement that each body will experience. These changes are derived from multiple factors, including non-exercise-induced activity thermogenesis (NEAT), emotional stress, temperature adaptions, physiological changes (for example, having a menstrual cycle), and recovery from injury or illness.

Finally, someone who has been subsisting on a very low daily calorie intake before commencing recovery from a malnourished state may need a lot more energy than will be conventionally accounted for. This "extra" energy will be needed to help restore the healthy function of numerous physiological processes, as well as makeup for hypermetabolism (a state in which metabolism will speed up to capture the increase in energy supplied), which may occur as part of this process.

CHAPTER 3

The Obesity hormonal mechanism

Hormones Trusted Sources are important substances that serve as chemical messengers in your body.

They facilitate nearly every bodily process, including metabolism trusted source, hunger, and fullness. Because of their association with appetite, some hormones also play a significant role in body weight trusted source

Starling's original definition of a hormone from 1905 was "a hormone is a substance produced by glands with internal secretion, which serve to carry signals through the blood to target organs". Today, this definition is understood to be lacking, but newer definitions also do not encompass the entire meaning of hormones as specific carriers of information. One main problem is that there is no delineation between hormones and other signaling molecules such as cytokines, growth factors, or autacoid compounds. It seems that a precise definition is not even possible, since some cytokines and growth factors, such as the cytokines erythropoietin, lipocalin-2, and asp rosin or fibroblast growth factor 23, act as hormones under certain conditions.

A system of glands, known as the endocrine system, secretes hormones into our bloodstream. The endocrine system works with the nervous system and the immune system to help our body cope with different events and stresses. Excesses or deficits of hormones can lead to obesity and, on the other hand, obesity can lead to changes in hormones.

Obesity and leptin

The hormone leptin is produced by fat cells and is secreted into our bloodstream. Leptin reduces a person's appetite by acting on specific centers of the brain to reduce the urge to eat. It also seems to control how the body manages its store of body fat.

Because leptin is produced by fat, leptin levels tend to be higher in people who are obese than in people of normal weight. However, despite having higher levels of this appetite-reducing hormone, people who are obese aren't as sensitive to the effects of leptin and, as a result, tend not to feel full during and after a meal. Ongoing research is looking at why leptin messages aren't getting through to the brain in people who are obese.

Obesity and insulin

Insulin, a hormone produced by the pancreas, is important for the regulation of carbohydrates and the metabolism of fat. Insulin stimulates glucose (sugar) uptake from the blood in tissues such as muscles, the liver, and fat. This is an important process to make sure that energy is available for everyday functioning and to maintain normal levels of circulating glucose.

In a person who is obese, insulin signals are sometimes lost and tissues are no longer able to control glucose levels. This can lead to the development of type II diabetes and metabolic syndrome.

Obesity and sex hormones

Body fat distribution plays an important role in the development of obesity-related conditions such as heart disease, stroke, and some forms of arthritis. Fat around our abdomen is a higher risk factor for disease than fat stored on our bottom, hips, and thighs. It seems that estrogens and androgens help to decide body fat distribution. Estrogens are sex hormones made by the ovaries in pre-menopausal women. They are responsible for prompting ovulation every menstrual cycle.

Men and postmenopausal women do not produce much estrogen in their testes (testicles) or ovaries. Instead, most of their estrogen is produced in their body fat, although at much lower amounts than what is produced in pre-menopausal ovaries. In younger men, androgens are produced at high levels in the testes. As a man gets older, these levels gradually decrease.

The changes with age in the sex hormone levels of both men and women are associated with changes in body fat distribution. While women of childbearing age tend to store fat in their lower body ('pear-shaped'), older men and postmenopausal women tend to increase the storage of fat around their abdomen ('apple-shaped'). Postmenopausal women who are taking estrogen supplements don't accumulate fat around their abdomen. Animal studies have also shown that a lack of estrogen leads to excessive weight gain.

Obesity and growth hormone

The pituitary gland in our brain produces growth hormone, which influences a person's height and helps build bone and muscle. Growth hormone also affects metabolism (the rate at which we burn kilojoules for energy). Researchers have found that growth hormone levels in people who are obese are lower than in people of normal weight.

Inflammatory factors and obesity

Obesity is also associated with low-grade chronic inflammation within the fat tissue. Excessive fat storage leads to stress reactions within fat cells, which in turn leads to the release of pro-inflammatory factors from the fat cells themselves and immune cells within the adipose (fat) tissue.

Obesity hormones as a risk factor for disease

Obesity is associated with an increased risk of several diseases, including cardiovascular disease, stroke, and several types of cancer, and with decreased longevity (shorter life span) and lower quality of life. For example, the increased production of estrogen in the fat of older women who are obese is associated with an increase in breast cancer risk, indicating that the source of estrogen production is important.

Behavior and obesity hormones

People who are obese have hormone levels that encourage the accumulation of body fat. It seems that behaviors such as overeating and lack of regular exercise, over time, 'reset' the processes that regulate appetite and body fat distribution to make the person physiologically more likely to gain weight. The body is always trying to maintain balance, so it resists any short-term disruptions such as crash dieting.

Various studies have shown that a person's blood leptin level drops after a low-kilojoule diet. Lower leptin levels may increase a person's appetite and slow down their metabolism. This may help to explain why crash dieters usually regain their lost weight. Leptin therapy may one day help dieters maintain their weight loss in the long term, but more research is needed before this becomes a reality.

There is evidence to suggest that long-term behavior changes, such as healthy eating and regular exercise, can re-train the body to shed excess body fat and keep it off. Studies have also shown that weight loss as a result of a healthy diet and exercise or bariatric surgery leads to improved insulin resistance, decreased inflammation, and beneficial modulation of obesity hormones. Weight loss is also associated with a decreased risk of developing heart disease, stroke, type II diabetes, and some cancers.

CHAPTER 4

How sugar causes obesity and abdominal fat accumulation.

The impact of sugar consumption on health continues to be a controversial topic. The objective of this review is to discuss the evidence and lack of evidence that allows the controversy to continue, and why resolution of the controversy is important.

There are plausible mechanisms and research evidence that support the suggestion that consumption of excess sugar promotes the development of cardiovascular disease (CVD) and type 2 diabetes (T2DM) both directly and indirectly. The direct pathway involves the unregulated hepatic uptake and metabolism of fructose, which leads to liver lipid accumulation, dyslipidemia, decreased insulin sensitivity, and increased uric acid levels. The epidemiological data suggest that these direct effects of fructose are pertinent to the consumption of fructose-containing sugars, sucrose, and HFCS, which are the predominant added sugars. Consumption of added sugar is associated with the development and/or prevalence of fatty liver, dyslipidemia, insulin resistance, hyperuricemia, cardiovascular disease, and type 2 diabetes, and many of these associations are independent of body weight gain or total energy intake. There are diet intervention studies in which human subjects exhibited increased circulating lipids and decreased insulin sensitivity when consuming high sugar compared with control diets. Most recently, our group has reported that supplementing the *ad libitum* diets of young adults with beverages containing 0, 10, 17.5, or 25% of daily energy requirement (Ereq) as high fructose corn syrup (HFCS) increased lipid/lipoprotein risk factors for cardiovascular disease (CVD) and uric acid in a dose-response manner. However, unconfounded studies conducted in healthy humans under a controlled, energy-balanced diet protocol that allow determination of the effects of sugar with diets that do not allow for body weight gain are lacking. Furthermore, there are recent reports that conclude that there are no adverse effects of consuming beverages containing up to 30% Ereq sucrose or HFCS, and the conclusions from several meta-analyses suggest that fructose has no specific adverse effects relative to any other carbohydrate.

Consumption of excess sugar may also promote the development of CVD and T2DM indirectly by causing increased body weight and fat gain, but this is also a topic of controversy. Mechanistically, it is plausible that fructose consumption causes increased energy intake and reduced energy expenditure due to its failure to stimulate leptin production. Functional magnetic resonance imaging of the brain demonstrates that the brain responds differently to fructose or fructose-containing sugars compared with glucose or aspartame. There are epidemiological studies that show sugar consumption is associated with body weight gain, and there are intervention studies in which consumption of *ad libitum* high sugar diets promoted increased body weight gain compared with consumption of *ad libitum* low sugar diets. However, there are no studies in which energy intake and weight gain were compared in subjects consuming high or low-sugar, blinded, *ad libitum* diets formulated to ensure both groups consumed a comparable macronutrient distribution and the same amounts of fiber. There is also little data to determine whether the form in which added sugar is consumed, as a beverage or as solid food, affects its potential to promote weight gain.

It will be very challenging to obtain the funding to conduct the clinical diet studies needed to address these evidence gaps, especially at the levels of added sugar that are commonly consumed. Yet, filling these evidence gaps may be necessary for supporting the policy changes that will help to turn the food environment into one that does not promote the development of obesity and metabolic disease.

The impact of added sugar consumption on health continues to be a controversial topic. In recent counterpoint reviews Bray and Popkin concluded that sugar-sweetened beverages play a role in the epidemics of obesity, metabolic syndrome, and fatty liver disease, while Kahn and Sievepiper concluded that there is no clear or convincing evidence that any dietary or added sugar has a unique or detrimental impact relative to any other source of calories on the development of obesity or diabetes. Therefore, the objective of this review is to discuss the evidence and lack of evidence that allows the controversy to continue. The evidence is divided into two topics: the direct and indirect effects of added sugar consumption on the development of metabolic disease. Studies needed to help resolve the controversy will be described, as well as the challenges involved in conducting these studies and the reasons they are needed.

The term added sugar consumption in this review refers to sugars not naturally occurring in foods and these consist mainly of sucrose and high fructose corn syrup (HFCS). It also refers to the sugars added to both beverages and solid foods, even though it cannot be assumed that sugar in solid foods and sugar in beverages have equivalent effects. This is discussed later in the review. The term metabolic disease is used to specifically refer to cardiovascular disease (CVD), type 2 diabetes (T2DM), and non-alcoholic fatty liver disease (NAFLD). Metabolic disease was chosen over metabolic syndrome because it is beyond the scope of this review to discuss in detail the evidence and mechanisms related to sugar and its associations with hypertension and central obesity.

The potential for both direct and indirect effects of added sugar consumption on metabolic disease

There is evidence to suggest that diets high in added sugar promote the development of metabolic diseases both directly and indirectly. Directly, the fructose component in sugar causes dysregulation of lipid and carbohydrate metabolism. Indirectly, sugar promotes positive energy balance, thus body weight and fat gain, which also cause dysregulation of lipid and carbohydrate metabolism. Due to the direct and indirect pathways, we have suggested that the risk for metabolic disease is exacerbated when added sugar is consumed with diets that allow for body weight and fat gain.

The prevalence of metabolic syndrome, cardiovascular disease, and type 2 diabetes are strongly associated with the presence of overweight and obesity. This has led to the widespread belief that diet impacts metabolic disease solely through the effects of excess body weight and fat. The sugar-related industries are campaigning vigorously to reinforce this belief and "educate" the public that the only dietary culprit is excess calories. However, if sugar consumption has direct effects that increase risk factors for metabolic disease in the absence of positive energy balance, this assertion is not true, and the public and health care providers need to be informed accordingly.

Plausible mechanisms by which consumption of sugar may independently contribute to the development of CVD and T2DM

Our group has reported that subjects consuming fructose-sweetened beverages for ten weeks exhibited increased de novo lipogenesis (DNL), dyslipidemia, and circulating uric acid levels and reduced fatty acid oxidation and insulin sensitivity, while subjects consuming glucose-sweetened beverages did not, despite comparable body weight gain. These results, our more recent results, and the results of many colleagues support the plausibility of the mechanisms

Chapter 5

The Obesity Solution Meal: How to Fight Sugar Cravings and Choose the Right Macronutrients

Beyond Willpower: Diet Quality and Quantity Matter

It's no secret that the *number* of calories people eat and drink has a direct impact on their weight: Consume the same number of calories that the body burns over time, and weight stays stable. Consume more than the body burns, weight goes up. Less, weight goes down. But what about the *type* of calories: Does it matter whether they come from specific nutrients- fat, protein, or carbohydrate? Specific whole grains or potato chips? Specific diets-the Mediterranean diet or the "Twinkie" diet? And what about *when* or *where* people consume their calories: Does eating breakfast make it easier to control weight? Does eating at fast-food restaurants make it harder?

There's ample research on foods and diet patterns that protect against heart disease, stroke, diabetes, and other chronic conditions. The good news is that many of the foods that help prevent disease also seem to help with weight control foods like whole grains, vegetables, fruits, and nuts. Many of the foods that increase disease risk-chief among them, refined grains and sugary drinks are also factors in weight gain. Conventional wisdom says that since a calorie is a calorie, regardless of its source, the best advice for weight control is simply to eat less and exercise more. Yet emerging research suggests that some foods and eating patterns may make it *easier* to keep calories in check, while others may make people more likely to overeat.

This article briefly reviews the research on dietary intake and weight control, highlighting diet strategies that also help prevent chronic disease.

Macronutrients and Weight: Do Carbs, Protein, or Fat Matter?

When people eat controlled diets in laboratory studies, the percentage of calories from fat, protein, and carbohydrates does not seem to matter for weight loss. In studies where people can freely choose what they eat, there may be some benefits to a higher protein, lower carbohydrate approach. For chronic disease prevention, though, the *quality and food sources* of these nutrients matter more than their relative *quantity* in the diet. And the latest research suggests that the same diet quality message applies to weight control.

Dietary Fat and Weight

Low-fat diets have long been touted as the key to a healthy weight and good health. But the evidence just isn't there: Over the past 30 years in the U.S., the percentage of calories from fat in people's diets has gone down, but obesity rates have skyrocketed. Carefully conducted clinical trials have found that following a low-fat diet does not make it any easier to lose weight than following a moderate- or high-fat diet. Study volunteers who follow moderate- or high-fat diets lose just as much weight, and in some studies a bit more, as those who follow low-fat diets. And when it comes to disease prevention, low-fat diets don't appear to offer any special benefits.

Part of the problem with low-fat diets is that they are often high in carbohydrates, especially from rapidly digested sources, such as white bread and white rice. And diets high in such foods increase the risk of weight gain, diabetes, and heart disease.

For good health, the type of fat people eat is far more important than the amount, and there's some evidence that the same may be true for weight control. In the Nurses' Health Study, for example, which followed 42,000 middle-aged and older women for eight years, increased consumption of unhealthy fats-trans fats, especially, but also saturated fats-was linked to weight gain, but increased consumption of healthy fats-monounsaturated and polyunsaturated fat-was not.

Protein and Weight

Read more about healthy proteins on The Nutrition Source

Higher protein diets seem to have some advantages for weight loss, though more so in short-term trials; in longer-term studies, high-protein diets seem to perform equally well as other types of diets. High-protein diets tend to be low in carbohydrates and high in fat, so it is difficult to tease apart the benefits of eating lots of protein from those of eating more fat or less carbohydrate. But there are a few reasons why eating a higher percentage of calories from protein may help with weight control:

· **More satiety:** People tend to feel fuller, on fewer calories, after eating protein than they do after eating carbohydrates or fat.

· **Greater thermic effect:** It takes more energy to metabolize and store protein than other macronutrients, and this may help people increase the energy they burn each day.

· **Improved body composition:** Protein seems to help people hang on to lean muscle during weight loss, and this, too, can help boost the energy-burned side of the energy balance equation.

Higher protein and lower carbohydrate diets improve blood lipid profiles and other metabolic markers, so they may help prevent heart disease and diabetes. But some high-protein foods are healthier than others: High intakes of red meat and processed meat are associated with an increased risk of heart disease, diabetes, and colon cancer.

Replacing red and processed meat with nuts, beans, fish, or poultry seems to lower the risk of heart disease and diabetes. And this diet strategy may help with weight control, too, according to a recent study from the Harvard School of Public Health. Researchers tracked the diet and lifestyle habits of 120,000 men and women for up to 20 years, looking at how small changes contributed to weight gain over time. People who ate more red and processed meat throughout the study gained more weight a pound extra every four years. People who ate more nuts throughout the study gained less weight a half pound less every four years.

Carbohydrates and Weight

Lower carbohydrate, higher protein diets may have some weight loss advantages in the short term. Yet when it comes to preventing weight gain and chronic disease, carbohydrate quality is much more important than carbohydrate quantity.

Read more about Carbohydrates on The Nutrition Source

Milled, refined grains and the foods made with them are white rice, white bread, white pasta, processed breakfast cereals, and the like-are rich in rapidly digested carbohydrates. So are potatoes and sugary drinks. The scientific term for this is that they have a high glycaemic index and glycaemic load. Such foods cause fast and furious increases in blood sugar and insulin that, in the short term, can cause hunger to spike and can lead to overeating and over the long term, increase the risk of weight gain, diabetes, and heart disease.

For example, in the diet and lifestyle change study, people who increased their consumption of French fries, potatoes and potato chips, sugary drinks, and refined grains gained more weight over time extra 3.4, 1.3, 1.0, and 0.6 pounds every four years, respectively. People who decreased their intake of these foods gained less weight.

Whole Grains, Fruits and Vegetables, and Weight

Read more about Whole grain on The Nutrition Source

Whole grains-whole wheat, brown rice, barley, and the like, especially in their less-processed forms digested more slowly than refined grains. So, they have a gentler effect on blood sugar and insulin, which may help keep hunger at bay. The same is true for most vegetables and fruits. These "slow carb" foods have bountiful benefits for disease prevention, and there's also evidence that they can help prevent weight gain.

Read more about vegetables and fruits on The Nutrition Source

The weight control evidence is stronger for whole grains than it is for fruits and vegetables. The most recent support comes from the Harvard School of Public Health diet and lifestyle change study: People who increased their intake of whole grains, whole fruits (not fruit juice), and vegetables throughout the 20-year study gained less weight-0.4, 0.5, and 0.2 pounds less every four years, respectively.

Of course, the calories from whole grains, whole fruits, and vegetables don't disappear. What's likely happening is that when people increase their intake of these foods, they cut back on calories from other foods. Fibre may be responsible for these foods' weight control benefits, since fiber slows digestion, helping to curb hunger. Fruits and vegetables are also high in water, which may help people feel fuller on fewer calories.

Nuts and Weight

Read more about nuts on The Nutrition Source

Nuts pack a lot of calories into a small package and are high in fat, so they were once considered taboo for dieters. As it turns out, studies find that eating nuts does not lead to weight gain and may instead help with weight control, perhaps because nuts are rich in protein and fiber, both of which may help people feel fuller and less hungry. People who regularly eat nuts are less likely to have heart attacks or die from heart disease than those who rarely eat them, which is another reason to include nuts in a healthy diet.

Dairy and Weight

Read more about calcium and milk on The Nutrition Source

The U.S. dairy industry has aggressively promoted the weight-loss benefits of milk and other dairy products, based largely on findings from short-term studies it has funded. However, a recent review of nearly 50 randomized trials finds little evidence that high dairy or calcium intake helps with weight loss. Similarly, most long-term follow-up studies have not found that dairy or calcium protect against weight gain and one study in adolescents found high milk intakes to be associated with increased body mass index.

One exception is the recent dietary and lifestyle change study from the Harvard School of Public Health, which found that people who increased their yogurt intake gained less weight; increases in milk and cheese intake, however, did not appear to promote weight loss or gain. The beneficial bacteria in yogurt may influence weight control, but more research is needed.

Chapter 6

Healthy Nutritional Supplements Programme

A diet and detox program called the Forever Living C9 Nutritional Cleansing Programme (formerly called the Clean 9) offers to help you lose weight quickly. The Forever Living C9 diet is one of many popular diets that promise fast weight loss.

However, many people who attempt fad diets fail to lose weight, and some of these diets are unhealthy to follow for an extended period. The Forever Living C9 diet is discussed in this article, along with what it is, what it involves, and whether it is worth attempting.

The Forever Living C9 diet: What is it?

The Forever Living C9 Nutritional Cleansing Programme, often known as Forever C9, is a 9-day detox diet for rapid weight loss. It was formerly known as the Clean 9 Diet. The utilization of meal replacement beverages and weight loss supplements is the main component of this low-calorie diet plan. It is the first of the Forever F.I.T. Program's three steps, which are as follows:

Weight management Forever C9 Nutritional Cleanse F15 V5 Sports Performance

The diet's proponents assert that it can aid in body cleansing, improve your appearance, make you feel lighter, and help you lose weight in just 9 days. You must acquire a Forever C9 diet pack from the Forever brand website or one of the participating. Kindly follow this link to purchase your order https://shopnow.foreverliving.com/USA/en-US/products?distribID=233100014389